KT-425-358

2100025226

E.L.R.S.

DIET AND NUTRITION
Fibre in Food
Miriam Moss

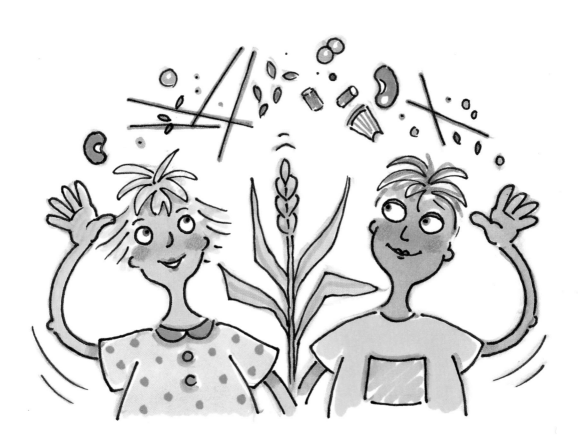

Wayland

S334882

641.1 [M]

DIET AND NUTRITION

Additives in Food
Vitamins in Food
Fibre in Food
Sugar in Food

Series editor: Deborah Elliott
Designer: Malcolm Walker
Cover design: Simon Balley
Artwork: John Yates
Cartoons: Maureen Jackson

First published in 1995 by
Wayland (Publishers) Limited
61 Western Road, Hove,
East Sussex, BN3 1JD, England

© Copyright 1995
Wayland (Publishers) Limited

Text is based on *Fibre* in the *Food Facts* series,
published in 1992

British Library Cataloguing in Publication Data
Moss, Miriam
  Fibre in food - (Diet and Nutrition series)
  I. Title   II. Series
  641.331
  ISBN 0 7502 1426 0

Typesetting by Kudos Editorial and Design Services
Printed and bound by Rotolito Lombarda s.p.a. Italy

Contents

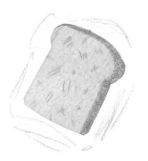

Fine fibre

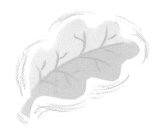

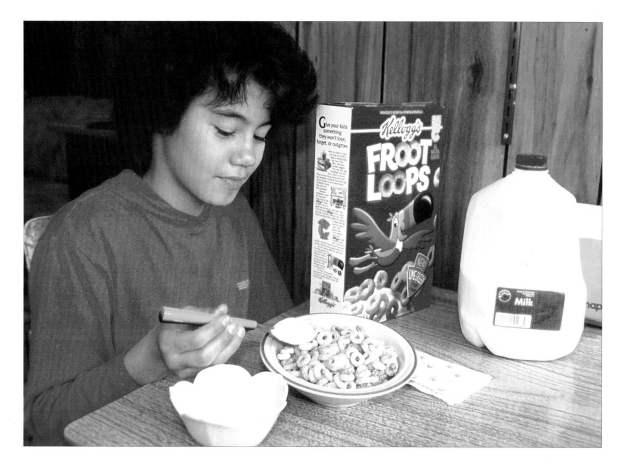

▲ *Look on your cereal box to see if it contains lots of fibre.*

Fibre is found in food. It is made of very fine threads. All living things are made up of millions of tiny cells. When you eat, your body turns the food cells into new body cells. The fibre in food helps your body to do this properly.

Foods that come from animals, such as meat, milk and eggs, do not have any fibre.

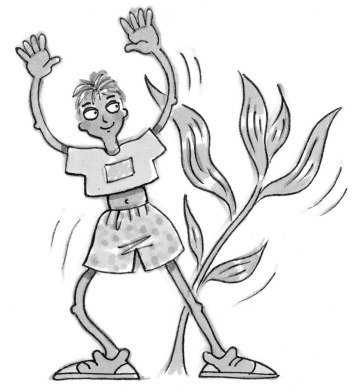

▼ *The rice, pasta, oats, flour and bread in this picture are full of fibre.*

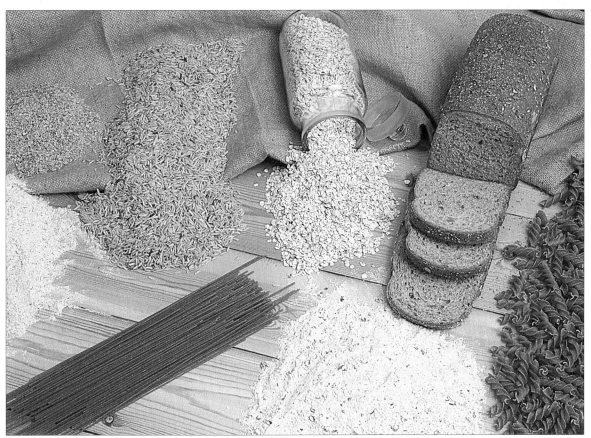

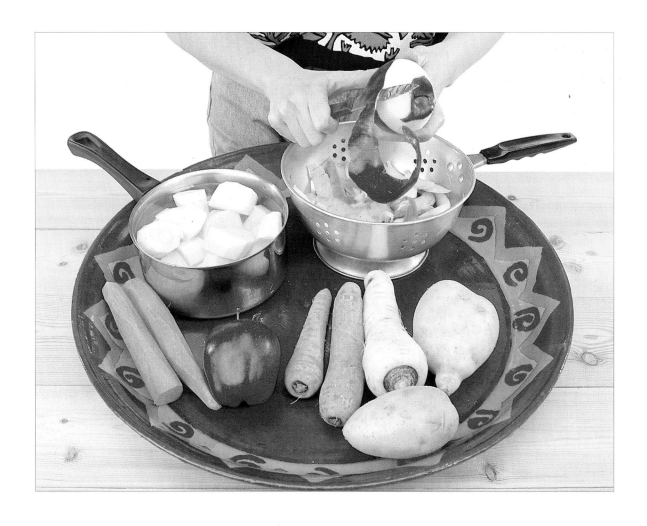

There is more fibre on the outside than on the inside of fruit and vegetables. If the outside is peeled away, the fibre is lost. Foods that have had their peel, skins or husks peeled away are known as refined or processed foods. They are low in fibre.

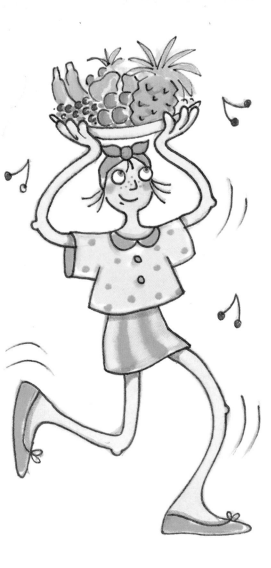

Raspberries and blackberries are very high in fibre. Have you noticed that they take longer to chew than strawberries? This is because they have more fibre.

► *Eating lots of fresh fruit gives you a healthy body and plenty of energy.*

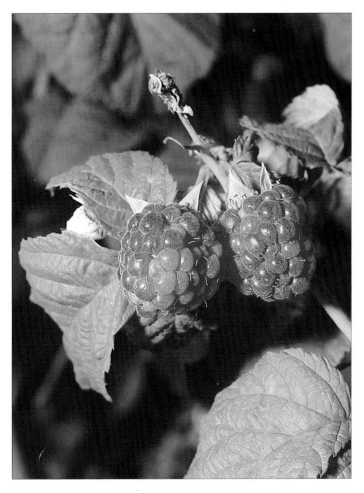

Spotting fibre

The way fruit feels and the time it takes to chew it are clues to how much fibre it contains. Check out some dried figs, apricots and prunes. They are all high in fibre. Cut them open and look at them through a magnifying glass. Can you see and feel the tiny threads? This is fibre.

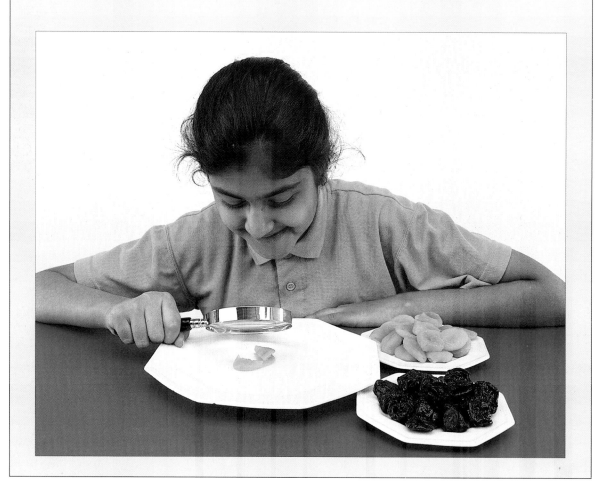

Nature's food

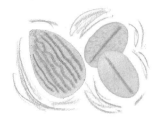

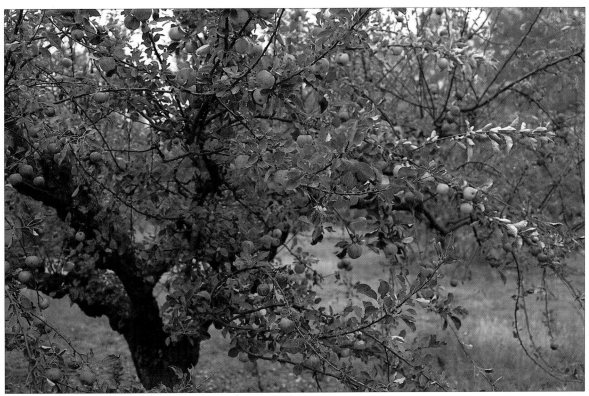

This apple tree, heavy with apples, stands in an orchard. Nowadays, most people buy their apples from a supermarket or grocery shop. It is easy to forget where our food actually comes from, and that nature provides everything we need for a healthy diet.

Fresh fruit

Autumn is the time of year when all the plants and trees in the countryside swell with fruits, nuts and berries. This basket contains gooseberries, hazelnuts, blackberries, blueberries, apples and rosehips. Make a list of other fruits, nuts or berries which ripen in autumn.

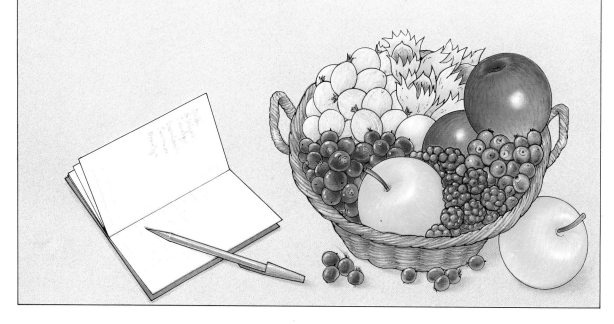

Corn ripens in the field and the farmers harvest the grain at the end of the summer. Bread made from flour using the whole grain, including the outside husk, is full of fibre. Grinding the tough grain into the soft flour we use to make bread used to be done using the power of the wind or of water.

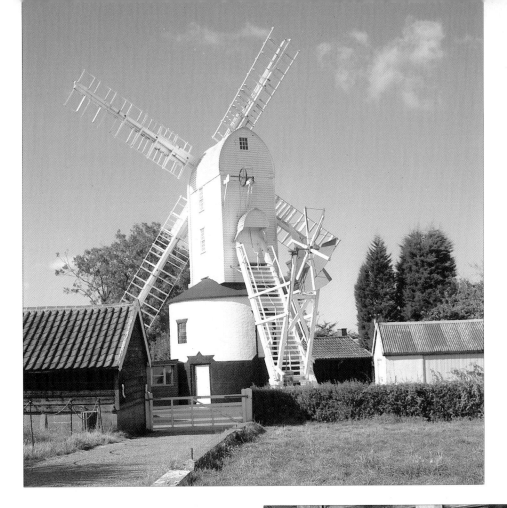

▲ *The wind turns the great sails of this windmill. They turn the heavy millstones inside which grind the grain into flour.*

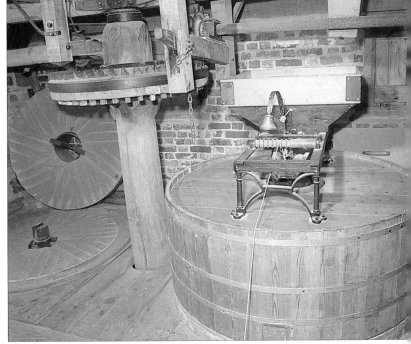

▶ *Falling river water outside this mill turns a huge wheel. The water wheel is joined to the wheels inside which grind the corn.*

The tasty sandwich in the photograph below is made with wholemeal bread. None of the husk has been removed. It contains at least twice as much fibre as the same sandwich made with white bread.

In ancient Egyptian and Roman times chalk was added to flour to make it white. Only rich people could afford to eat the expensive bread made from white flour. Poor people ate dark wholemeal bread which was much better for them anyway!

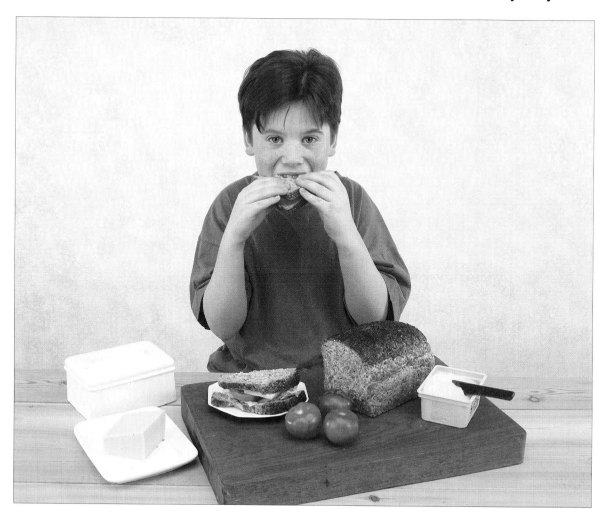

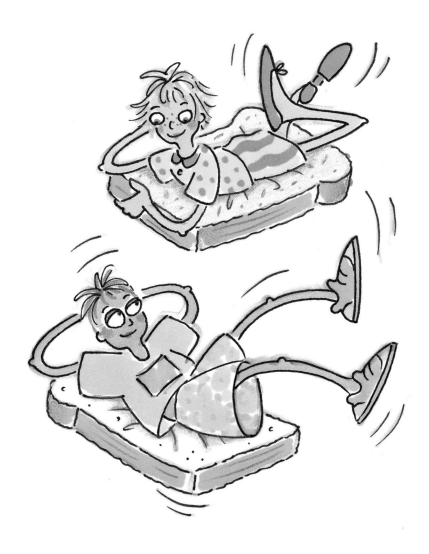

About 150 years ago, mills were built which could make white bread cheaply. Poor people who ate a lot of this cheap white bread suddenly lost a lot of fibre from their diet.

White sugar and white rice are refined foods. Unrefined sugar made from sugar beet or cane is brown. White rice has had the healthy outer layer polished off.

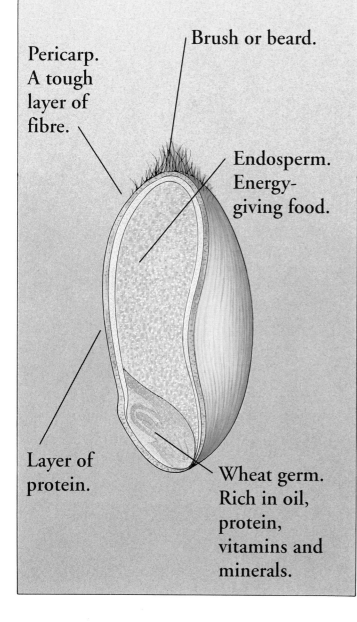

Inside a grain

If you cut a grain of wheat in half and looked at it under a magnifying glass this is what you might see.

Brush or beard.

Pericarp.
A tough
layer of
fibre.

Endosperm.
Energy-
giving food.

Layer of
protein.

Wheat germ.
Rich in oil,
protein,
vitamins and
minerals.

There are many reasons why so many people choose to eat refined food even though so much of the goodness is wasted.

Refined food is quick to prepare and can be stored for longer than fresh food.

If you fill your cupboards with refined food you don't need to shop every day.

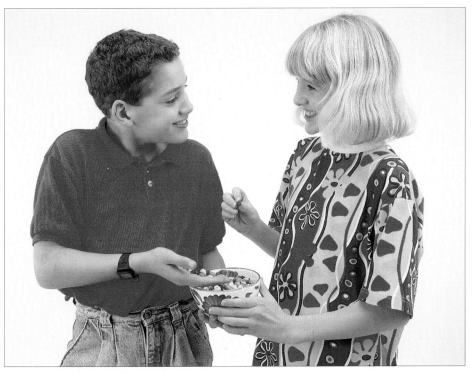

Nuts and raisins are much better for you than crisps. They are full of fibre.

A packet of crisps is much more expensive than the same weight of potatoes. You are paying the person who makes the crisp for peeling the potatoes (and removing all the fibre), and for adding fat, salt and chemical flavourings, which are all bad for you!

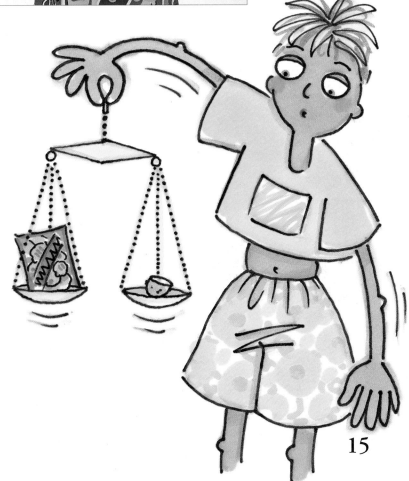

15

Making wholemeal bread

Make sure you have an adult to help you.
You will need:

1.5 kg wholemeal flour	large mixing bowl
1 tablespoon of salt	measuring jug
60 g fresh yeast or 30 g dried yeast	tablespoon
1 litre lukewarm water	wooden spoon
1 tablespoon of honey	three 1 kg loaf tins

1. Put the flour and the salt in the bowl.
2. Mix the yeast and the honey with half of the water.
3. When the mixture begins to bubble, make a space in the middle of the flour and mix in the yeast, honey and water.
4. Add the rest of the water, a little at a time, as you knead the dough. It should be spongy but not wet.
5. Leave the dough in its bowl in a warm place until it doubles in size. Then knead it again for a few minutes.
6. Divide the dough into three. Put the dough in the three loaf tins. Bake at the top of the oven at 350 ^{0}C, gas mark 7, for 35-40 minutes. When the loaves are cooked they sound hollow if you tap them.

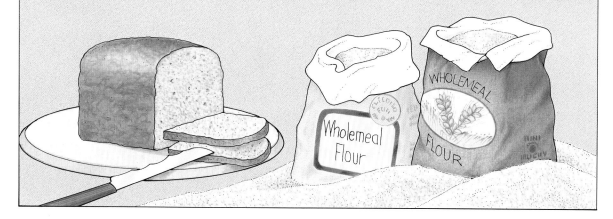

Looking after your body

Food is chewed into smaller pieces in your mouth. It goes down your throat into your stomach, where strong juices work it into a smooth paste.

This paste is squeezed into the small intestine and passes through the wall into the blood. It travels around your body repairing cells and giving you energy.

The bulky lump of waste left over in your large intestine is pushed out into the toilet.

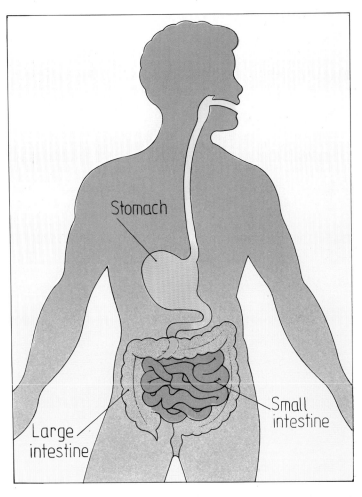

Stomach

Large intestine

Small intestine

▲ *Fibre helps with digestion. This diagram shows the parts of your body which digest food.*

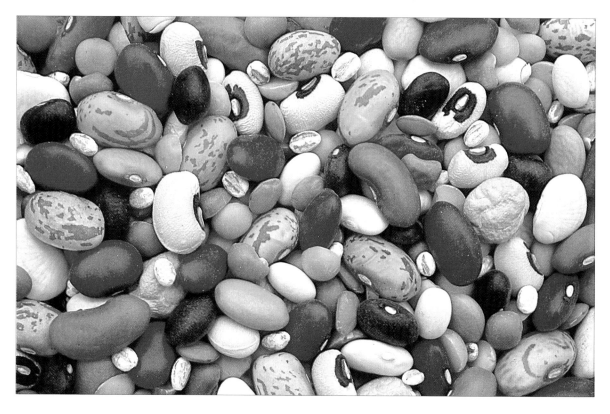

▲ *Beans and pulses are full of fibre.*

People who eat lots of fibre digest their food and get rid of their waste quickly and easily. Beans and pulses are full of fibre and are very good for digestion. They come in lots of different colours, shapes and tastes.

It is much healthier for you to get rid of your waste quickly than for it to stay in your body a long time.

Scientists have measured the time it takes for food to pass right through people's bodies.

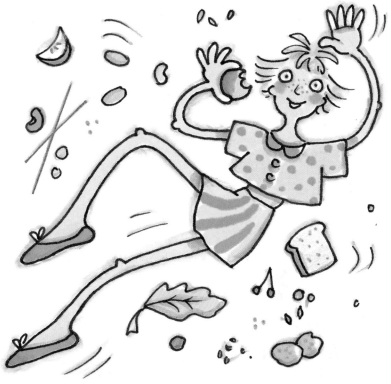

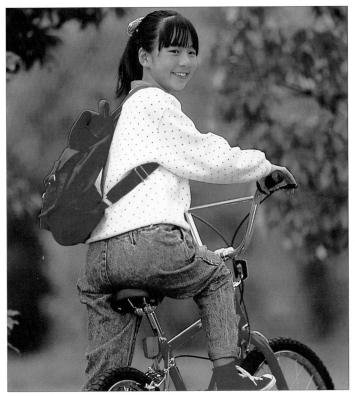

It only takes one and a half days for people who eat lots of fibre. For people who eat too many refined foods, it can take up to two weeks!

◄ *Exercise also helps you to digest food. Try to do at least half an hour's exercise each day.*

▼ *This freshly cooked curry is perfect for a healthy diet. The rice and chopped vegetables are full of fibre, vitamins and minerals.*

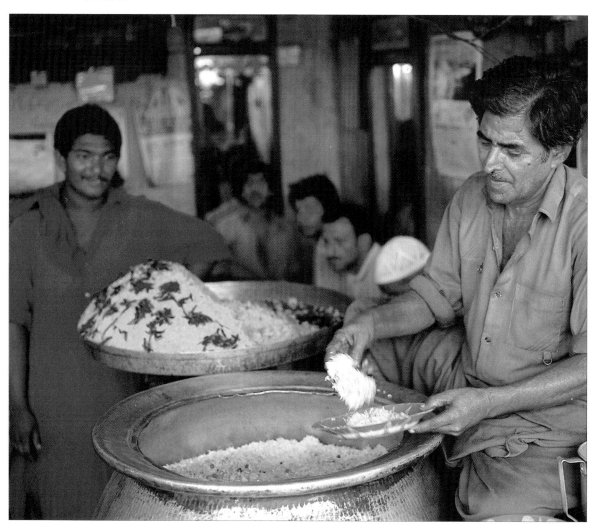

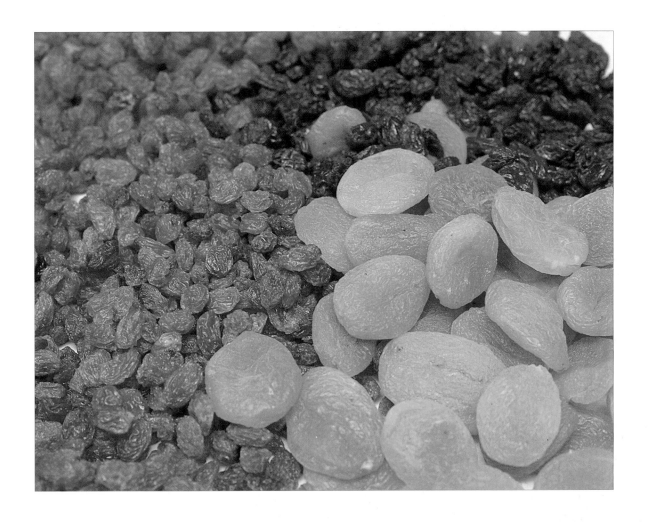

Dried fruits such as currants, sultanas and apricots (above) are delicious and very high in fibre. They make a very good snack if you are feeling hungry between meals. It's easier than you think to change your diet to include more fibre!

Eat more fibre!

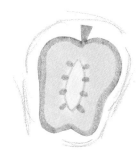

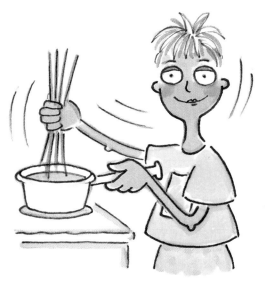

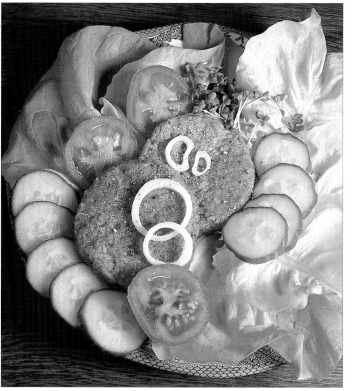

▼ *What about a high fibre veggie burger? Go on, try one.*

Look after your body and swap to high fibre foods! Try eating wholemeal bread instead of white bread. Choose brown rice instead of white. Eat wholemeal pasta – it takes longer to cook but it tastes better. Pastry, cakes and biscuits are delicious made from wholemeal flour.

Brown rice Pilaf

Try making this quick, delicious fibre-full meal. Make sure you have an adult to help you.

You will need:

A bunch of spring onions 150 g brown rice   wooden spoon
1 small onion   2 teaspoons oil   non-stick frying pan
1 red pepper   salt and pepper   knife
1 green pepper   2 teaspoons butter
100 g mushrooms $\frac{1}{2}$ litre of water
1 carrot

1. Chop the vegetables into very small pieces.
2. Fry the vegetables in the oil and butter for five minutes and add salt and pepper.
3. Add the rice and fry for one minute.
4. Add water and leave to simmer for 40 minutes.

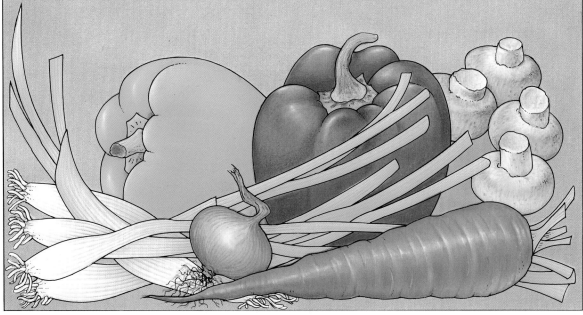

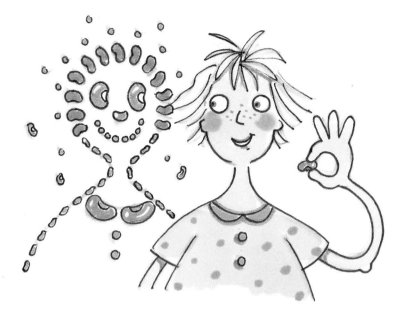

▼ Did you know that soya beans contain the same amount of protein as the same weight of steak – and they are high in fibre, too.

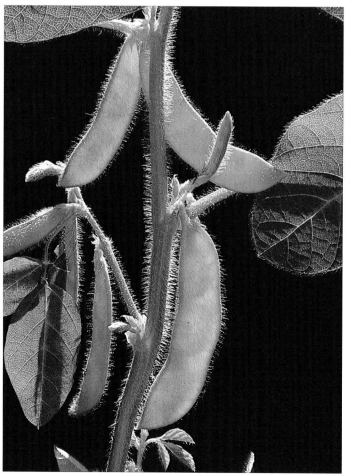

Some people worry that if they don't eat animal products like meat and cheese they will miss out on the protein these foods contain. But peas and beans contain lots of protein and lots of fibre, too!

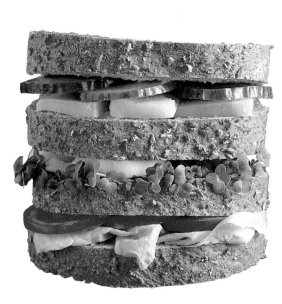

▲ *Make sure your sandwiches contain lots of different fibre-full foods. Try experimenting by mixing different tastes in lots of layers!*

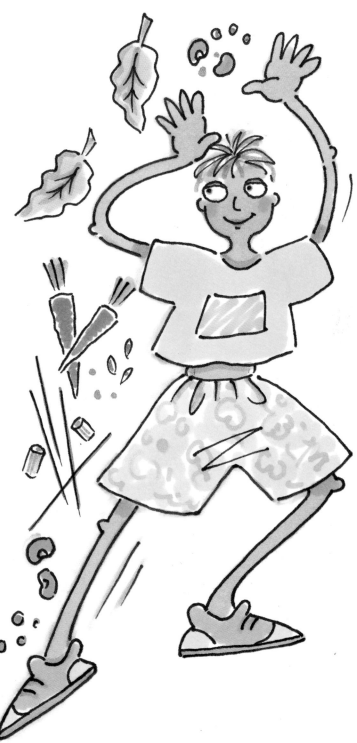

▼ *Check out the amount of fibre in these foods.*

Amount of fibre in 100g of some foods

Almonds		14·3g	Fried egg		0· g
Apples		1·5g	Grapefruit		0·6g
Apricots (dried)		24·0g	Muesli (average mixture)		7·4g
Bacon		0· g	Oranges		1·5g
Baked beans		7·3g	Pasta (white)		0· g
Bran		44·0g	Pasta (wholemeal)		10· g
Bread (white)		2·7g	Potatoes (cooked in skin)		2·5g
Bread (wholemeal)		8·5g	Raspberries		7·4g
Cornflakes		1· g	Sausages		0· g
			Weetabix		12·7g

Two breakfasts

Look at these two breakfasts. Which one do your think has the most fibre?

Breakfast One
Orange juice
Fried egg, bacon and sausage

Two slices of white toast with butter and marmalade

Breakfast Two
Half a grapefruit
Weetabix or muesli with yoghurt
Two slices of wholemeal toast with raspberry jam

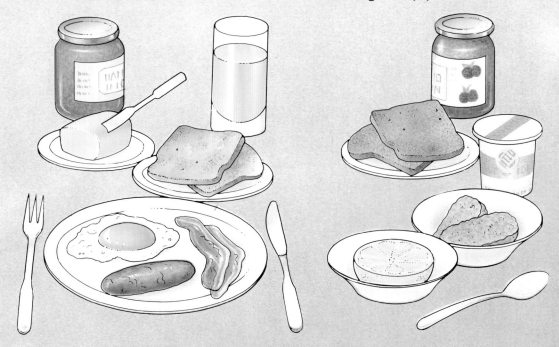

This breakfast contains about 2 g of fibre.

This breakfast contains about 12 g of fibre.

Fibre detectives

The labels on cereal, rice and pasta packets often tell you how much fibre is found in 100 g of the food.

Collect together some different foods and keep their labels.
Then weigh out 100 g of the food on a pair of sales.
Now ask a friend to guess (without looking at the food label) how much fibre is in each 100 g.
Score points for a close guess.

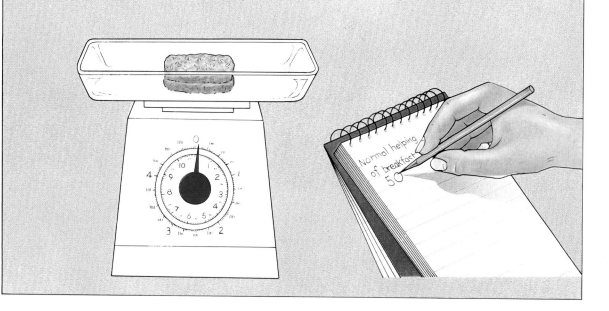

Bran contains more fibre than any other food, but it is quite hard to eat on its own. Try making your own breakfast cereal. Choose your favourite nuts and fresh and dried fruit, and add oats and bran. You can mix in the milk the night before to soften the oats if you prefer. Or you can add the milk just before you eat it for a crunchier breakfast. Why not give your recipe its own special name?

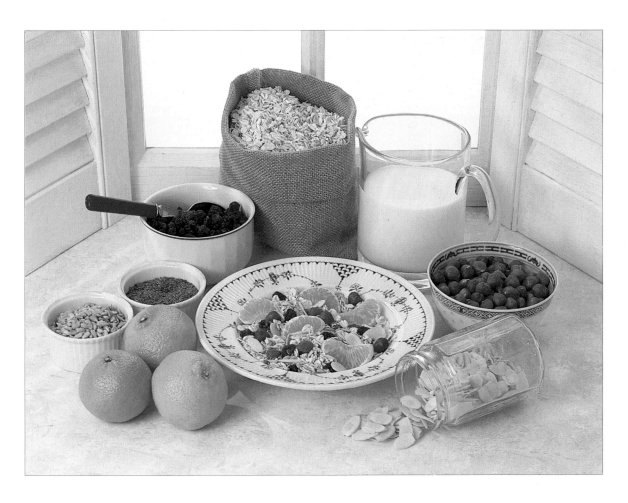

Glossary

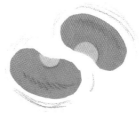

bran   Part of the outside skin of cereals. Bran contains a lot of fibre.

cells   Tiny parts of living things which are too small to see without a microscope.

cereals   Grains such as wheat and barley and the foods made from them.

diet   All the food a person eats.

digested   To have taken in what the body needs from the food eaten.

knead   To pound and fold bread dough.

protein   Body-building food that helps your body to grow.

yeast   Something used to make bread rise.

Books to read

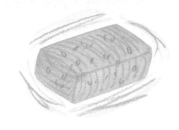

Diet by Brian Ward (Franklin Watts, 1991)

Food For Thought by Gill Standring (A & C Black, 1990)

Fruit by Miriam Moss (A & C Black, 1991)

Healthy Eating by Wayne Jackman (Wayland, 1990)

Beans by Terry Jennings (A & C Black, 1990)

Picture acknowledgements
Aspect 9; Cash 11 (top), 22, 25; Cephas 20; Chapel Studio 5, 6, 8, 11 (bottom), 12, 15, 21; Bruce Coleman 7, 24; Jeff Greenberg 4; Tony Stone19; Zefa 18, 29. The cover was photographed by Zul Mukhida and styled by Zoe Hargreaves.

Index

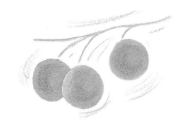